Preventive Measures and Protective Processes

A Practical Framework For Healthcare Safety

Everett Langley Hadley,Prescott

Table of Contents

1 Introduction to Healthcare Safety

Healthcare safety isn't just about avoiding accidents; it's about creating a system where harm is minimized, and well-being is prioritized. It's a proactive approach, anticipating potential problems and implementing measures to prevent them before they even arise. This fundamentally changes the healthcare experience, transforming it from a potentially risky environment into a safe and supportive one. Think of it like building a house - you wouldn't start constructing without blueprints and safety regulations, would you? Healthcare safety demands the same meticulous planning.

Effective risk assessment is paramount. It involves systematically identifying potential hazards, analyzing their likelihood and severity, and subsequently developing strategies to mitigate those risks. This isn't a one-time process; it's an ongoing cycle of evaluation, adjustment, and improvement. Regular review and updates are essential to adapt to changing circumstances and new information. For instance, a hospital might conduct a thorough risk assessment of its surgical unit, analyzing the possibility of surgical site infections, medication errors, or falls. The results would then inform the development of protocols to reduce those risks. Remember, proactive risk management is more cost-effective in the long run than reacting to incidents after they occur.

Consider the human element. Healthcare is a people-centric industry. The success of safety initiatives greatly depends on the active participation and commitment of every individual involved. From doctors and nurses to administrative staff and support personnel, everyone plays a crucial role. Effective communication is essential for coordinating efforts, ensuring that everyone is aware of their responsibilities, and fostering a collaborative culture of safety. Regular training and education on safety protocols are key to maintaining competency and promoting a shared understanding of best practices. Open communication channels are also vital for reporting near misses and incidents, allowing for prompt corrective actions.

A culture of safety isn't simply a set of rules; it's a mindset. It's about creating an environment where individuals feel comfortable reporting errors or concerns without fear of retribution. This requires fostering open communication, mutual respect, and a commitment to continuous learning. This isn't about blaming individuals; it's about identifying system-level issues and implementing improvements to prevent future occurrences. Imagine a team where everyone feels empowered to speak up if they see something unsafe. That's the power of a safety culture. This fosters trust and promotes a sense of collective responsibility for patient safety.

Implementing safety measures requires resources. This might include financial investment in equipment, training programs, or technological solutions. However, it's crucial to prioritize cost-effectiveness, selecting the most impactful interventions that provide the greatest return on investment. A hospital might invest in new fall prevention equipment, resulting in a significant reduction in fall-related injuries, justifying the financial commitment. The return on investment is not just monetary; it includes improved patient outcomes and a more positive work environment.

Technological advancements play a significant role in enhancing healthcare safety. Electronic health records can reduce medication errors by providing real-time alerts and preventing medication interactions. Telemedicine can enhance access to care and monitoring, especially for patients in remote areas. Advanced monitoring systems can detect potential problems early, enabling prompt intervention. However, it is essential to remember that technology is a tool; it's the human element that remains central to providing safe and effective care. Technology can assist, but human judgement and compassion must never be neglected.

Compliance with regulations is non-negotiable. Healthcare organizations are bound by various regulations and standards aimed at maintaining safety. Adherence to these regulations not only protects patients but also safeguards the reputation and legal standing of the healthcare provider. This includes compliance with infection control protocols, medication safety guidelines, and emergency response plans. Regular audits and inspections ensure compliance and highlight areas needing improvement. Consistent adherence builds trust and demonstrates a commitment to quality and safety.

Beyond regulatory compliance, continuous improvement is a journey, not a destination. Regular data collection and analysis identify areas needing improvement, and the findings should guide the development and implementation of targeted interventions. This iterative process ensures ongoing enhancement of safety measures and allows organizations to adapt to evolving challenges. For example, tracking the frequency of medication errors can reveal patterns and trends, enabling the development of strategies to reduce those errors. Continuous improvement requires a commitment to learning from both successes and failures. Every near miss, every incident, offers valuable insights that can prevent future problems.

1.1 Defining Healthcare Safety

Healthcare safety isn't simply the absence of harm; it's a proactive, multifaceted approach to minimizing risks and maximizing positive patient outcomes. It encompasses a complex interplay of factors, including the physical environment, medical procedures, staff training, and even the overall organizational culture. This holistic view is critical for creating truly safe healthcare environments.

Effective healthcare safety demands a comprehensive risk assessment process. This isn't a one-time event but an ongoing cycle of identification, analysis, and mitigation. We must consistently identify potential hazards - from slips and falls to medication errors to infection outbreaks - and then analyze the likelihood and severity of these hazards. This analysis informs the development of effective mitigation strategies, which might include new protocols, equipment upgrades, or staff training initiatives. The continuous nature of this process ensures that our safety measures remain relevant and effective.

Consider the impact of a single medication error. The consequences can range from minor discomfort to severe complications, even death. A thorough understanding of medication safety procedures, including proper administration, dosage calculations, and patient verification, is not optional; it's fundamentally vital to minimizing errors. Furthermore, robust systems for reporting and analyzing medication errors are crucial. This data helps pinpoint weaknesses in our processes and informs preventative measures. Open communication about medication errors, without blame, is key to learning from mistakes and implementing improvements.

Patient safety also extends beyond medication. Falls are a major concern for hospitalized patients, often leading to injuries and prolonged recovery times. Comprehensive fall risk assessments, preventative measures like bed alarms and assistive devices, and staff training on safe patient handling techniques significantly reduce fall-related incidents. Remember, it's not just about reacting to falls; it's about actively preventing them through meticulous planning and proactive intervention.

Similarly, pressure ulcers are a serious and often preventable complication. Regular skin assessments, proper positioning techniques, and the use of pressure-relieving surfaces play a crucial role in minimizing pressure ulcer development. Consistent monitoring and proactive intervention are essential components of effective pressure ulcer prevention strategies. The cost of treating pressure ulcers, both financially and emotionally, is substantial; therefore, their prevention represents a significant return on investment in safety initiatives.

Beyond individual patient risks, healthcare safety also involves creating a culture of safety within the entire organization. This requires fostering open communication, encouraging reporting of near misses and errors without fear of retribution, and promoting continuous learning. Staff training, regular safety audits, and leadership commitment are all integral to building a strong safety culture. A culture where safety is prioritized at every level isn't just a good idea; it's a necessity for providing high-quality care.

Effective emergency preparedness is another critical aspect of healthcare safety. This includes having robust disaster plans, well-defined code response protocols, and reliable communication systems. Regular drills and training exercises ensure that staff are prepared to respond effectively to various emergencies. Emergency preparedness isn't a luxury; it's a fundamental responsibility that directly impacts patient safety and staff well-being, preparing us for the unexpected.

The pursuit of healthcare safety is a continuous journey, not a destination. It requires constant vigilance, ongoing education, and a commitment to improvement. By prioritizing safety in all aspects of healthcare delivery, from basic hygiene practices to sophisticated technology integration, we can create environments that protect patients and staff alike. It's not just about avoiding harm; it's about actively fostering a safe and effective healthcare system. This continuous pursuit for improvement means regularly reviewing and updating our procedures, adapting to new technologies, and learning from past experiences. Only through this sustained commitment can we truly define and achieve comprehensive healthcare safety. Therefore, ongoing evaluation and adaptation are critical components in creating an environment that prioritizes safety above all else. This dedication to continuous improvement and refinement is the cornerstone of ensuring a consistently safe healthcare environment.

1.2 Risk Assessment Basics

Understanding risk is paramount in healthcare. It's not just about identifying potential hazards; it's about proactively mitigating them before they cause harm. This involves a systematic approach, not guesswork. We must move beyond reactive responses to accidents and embrace a culture of anticipating and preventing them. A proactive approach saves lives and resources.

Effective risk assessment starts with identification. This requires a multidisciplinary approach. Nurses, doctors, technicians, administrators—everyone has a role to play in spotting potential risks. Look at your environment; consider the patient population; analyze procedures. Is there inadequate lighting increasing fall risks? Are there medication storage issues? What about communication breakdowns during emergencies? Thoroughly document all observations, no matter how small they seem. A seemingly minor detail can be a critical piece of the puzzle. Every aspect needs meticulous consideration.

Next, analyze the identified risks. This goes beyond simple identification. We must determine the likelihood of each risk occurring and the severity of the potential consequences. For instance, a minor equipment malfunction might be unlikely but could have severe consequences if it happened during a critical procedure. Use a standardized risk assessment matrix to help quantify these factors. This methodical approach provides a consistent framework for prioritizing actions. A simple color-coded system can be very effective.

After analysis, we prioritize. Not all risks are created equal. Focus on those with the highest likelihood and greatest potential impact. Develop a clear action plan for each prioritized risk. Who is responsible? What needs to be done? When must it be completed? Assign responsibilities and deadlines to ensure accountability and timely action. Remember, an effective action plan should be dynamic and adaptable to changes in the healthcare environment. Consistent monitoring and adjustment are key.

Implementing the action plan is crucial, but equally crucial is monitoring its effectiveness. Regularly review the controls implemented. Are they working as intended? Are they adequate to mitigate the identified risks? If not, make adjustments accordingly. This cycle of risk assessment, analysis, prioritization, implementation, and monitoring is continuous. It's not a one-time event; it's an ongoing process essential for maintaining a safe healthcare environment. Continuous improvement is the ultimate goal.

Effective risk communication is also vital. Keep all stakeholders informed of identified risks, implemented controls, and monitoring results. This transparency builds trust and promotes a culture of safety. Regular staff training, open communication channels, and prompt reporting of near misses help foster a collaborative effort. The entire team must be on board to succeed in maintaining a safe healthcare environment for everyone. It is a shared responsibility.

Finally, remember that risk assessment is not about eliminating all risk, which is realistically impossible. The goal is to minimize risks to an acceptable level while continuing to provide high-quality care. It's about managing risk effectively and responsibly. This involves making informed decisions based on a thorough understanding of the risks and potential impacts. This balance between safety and service provision is critical to success.

Don't underestimate the power of involving staff at all levels in the risk assessment process. Their insights, based on their daily experiences, are invaluable. Create a culture where reporting of near misses is encouraged, without fear of retribution. Analyzing near misses can help pinpoint potential vulnerabilities before they cause accidents. This proactive approach fosters a safer, more efficient healthcare setting. Constant vigilance is crucial.

2 Infection Prevention and Control

Effective hand hygiene is the cornerstone of infection prevention. Washing hands thoroughly with soap and water for at least 20 seconds, or using an alcohol-based hand rub when soap and water aren't available, is crucial before and after patient contact, before and after donning and doffing personal protective equipment (PPE), and after touching potentially contaminated surfaces. Remember, consistent hand hygiene significantly reduces the transmission of many pathogens. This seemingly simple practice is demonstrably effective in preventing healthcare-associated infections. The World Health Organization (WHO) provides detailed guidelines, which should be readily accessible to all healthcare professionals, and regular training should be mandatory to ensure proficiency and adherence. Compliance monitoring, and regular feedback, are essential elements of successful hand hygiene programs, helping identify areas needing improvement and reinforcing best practices. Ignoring this fundamental aspect of infection control is irresponsible, risking patient and staff safety.

Proper use of PPE is paramount. This includes gloves, gowns, masks, eye protection, and respirators, each with specific applications. Gloves should be worn for all patient contact, regardless of the perceived risk, and changed between patients. Gowns are necessary when there's a risk of splashing or spraying of bodily fluids. Masks protect against airborne pathogens, while eye protection shields the eyes from splashes. Respirators, such as N95 masks, provide greater protection against airborne pathogens, and their proper use requires specific training. Knowing when to use each type of PPE and understanding the correct donning and doffing procedures are vital to prevent self-contamination and cross-contamination. Regular audits of PPE usage and adherence to protocols are essential, ensuring staff are correctly utilizing PPE and appropriate resources are available. Failure to utilize PPE correctly can result in serious consequences, for both patients and healthcare workers.

Environmental cleaning plays a significant role in infection control. Regular cleaning and disinfection of frequently touched surfaces, such as doorknobs, bedrails, and equipment, using appropriate disinfectants, is essential. Hospitals and clinics must develop and meticulously follow standardized cleaning protocols, including detailed schedules and specific cleaning agents. These protocols must address all areas of the facility, including patient rooms, common areas, and equipment. Effective cleaning requires attention to detail, ensuring thorough coverage of all surfaces. Regular monitoring and evaluation of cleaning practices, perhaps through environmental testing, can identify areas of weakness and improve effectiveness. This approach helps prevent the buildup of pathogens and minimizes the risk of transmission. Investing in effective cleaning supplies and providing sufficient training to cleaning staff are crucial aspects of a comprehensive infection control program.

Beyond these fundamental practices, implementing a robust infection control program requires a multi-faceted approach. This involves regular staff training and education, clear protocols and guidelines, thorough investigation and management of outbreaks, as well as ongoing monitoring and evaluation. Surveillance systems should be in place to track infection rates and identify potential outbreaks promptly. Immediate responses should be prepared and implemented in case of suspected infection spread. Effective communication between staff members is crucial for successful infection prevention and control. Regular review and updating of infection prevention and control policies ensure that they remain relevant and effective in addressing evolving challenges and improving healthcare safety. These components work in harmony, reducing the risk of healthcare-associated infections.

Regular staff training is absolutely essential. Healthcare professionals require ongoing education about infection prevention and control practices. This education should include hands-on training, regular refresher courses, and readily available resources. Training sessions should cover all aspects of infection control, emphasizing the importance of each practice and its role in overall patient safety. Staff feedback and active participation in training improve understanding and retention of key information. Continuous monitoring of staff adherence to infection control procedures is also crucial. This helps identify areas where additional training might be needed or where protocols could be improved. Regular assessment and feedback are integral parts of successful infection control training, improving overall compliance and promoting a culture of safety. A commitment to ongoing learning and improvement is imperative for maintaining high standards of infection control.

2.1 Hand Hygiene Techniques

Effective hand hygiene is paramount in healthcare, preventing the transmission of infections and safeguarding both patients and healthcare workers. This involves more than just a quick rinse; it's a meticulous process demanding attention to detail and consistent practice. Remember, even seemingly minor lapses can have significant consequences.

Proper handwashing begins with wetting your hands under clean, running water—ideally warm, but cold water works too, especially in resource-limited settings. Then, apply enough soap to cover all surfaces, creating a lather. This lather should be thorough, reaching between fingers, under nails, and around wrists. Don't rush this step; take at least 20 seconds—the time it takes to sing "Happy Birthday" twice—to ensure complete coverage. Scrub vigorously, removing dirt, grime, and transient microorganisms. This is not merely a cosmetic exercise; it's a crucial step in pathogen removal. Rinsing thoroughly is just as vital, eliminating any soap residue that could irritate the skin.

Hand sanitizers, containing at least 60% alcohol, provide an excellent alternative when soap and water aren't readily available. However, they are not a universal substitute. Visible soil requires soap and water pre-cleaning; sanitizers can't penetrate grime and will not effectively kill pathogens. Apply the sanitizer to the palms of your hands, rubbing it thoroughly across all surfaces. Continue rubbing until your hands are completely dry, ensuring the alcohol has time to evaporate and complete its germicidal action. The drying process itself helps remove pathogens mechanically. It's also important to note that prolonged use of alcohol-based sanitizers can dry out the skin leading to cracks, so consider using a moisturizing lotion afterwards. This helps maintain the integrity of your skin barrier, reducing the risk of infection.

Beyond the mechanics, understanding the 'why' behind hand hygiene is equally important. Healthcare settings are teeming with microorganisms, some harmless, many pathogenic. Patients are particularly vulnerable; their immune systems may be compromised, making them susceptible to infections that a healthy individual might easily fight off. Hand hygiene acts as a crucial barrier, breaking the chain of infection. It prevents the transfer of pathogens from one patient to another, from a healthcare worker to a patient, or vice-versa. The concept is simple, yet its consistent practice forms the cornerstone of infection control.

Consider the context of each hand hygiene event. Before touching a patient, you are protecting them from potentially harmful bacteria from your skin, for instance, from an encounter with another patient or a contaminated surface. After touching a patient, you prevent the transmission of potentially harmful pathogens from the patient to another patient, healthcare professional, or environmental surface. Before performing an aseptic procedure, you maintain a sterile field, minimizing the chances of introducing infection. After touching a patient's surroundings (bedrails, call bells etc.), you prevent spreading any potential pathogens you might have inadvertently touched, ensuring both your and your patient's safety.

Proper hand hygiene isn't just about individual actions; it's about creating a culture of safety within the healthcare environment. This requires clear protocols, readily available supplies, and consistent reinforcement of these practices. Regular training and audits can ensure compliance, and highlighting success stories can encourage everyone to maintain high hygiene standards. Creating posters and visual cues emphasizing the five moments for hand hygiene—before patient contact, before a clean/aseptic procedure, after body fluid exposure/risk, after patient contact, and after touching patient surroundings—can serve as visual reminders. Regular feedback and education are vital for sustaining high standards and preventing complacency, which can lead to lapses in hygiene. Remember, healthcare is a team effort, and everyone plays a role in maintaining a safe and infection-free environment. Every handwashing event is an opportunity to safeguard the health of your patients, your colleagues, and yourself. It's a simple act with powerful implications. It's an investment in safety, an investment in lives.

2.2 Personal Protective Equipment (PPE)

Choosing the right PPE is crucial; it's not a one-size-fits-all situation. Consider the specific hazard you're facing. Are you dealing with a potential bloodborne pathogen exposure? A respiratory illness? A chemical spill? Each scenario demands different protective gear. Understanding the risk is the first step toward effective protection. Failing to use the correct PPE increases the risk of exposure significantly, potentially leading to serious health consequences for yourself and your patients. This isn't simply about following protocol; it's about safeguarding your well-being and contributing to a safer healthcare environment.

Proper donning and doffing procedures are essential to prevent contamination. These steps should be meticulously followed, adhering to the established protocols for each type of PPE. A common mistake is neglecting the proper order of donning and doffing, increasing the chance of cross-contamination. Remember, this is not just about you; protecting your colleagues and patients is equally important. Consistent and precise adherence to the procedures is non-negotiable for maintaining a high standard of safety. Rushing these processes invites preventable infections and compromises the safety of all involved.

Gloves are the most frequently used PPE item, protecting your hands from contact with bodily fluids and other potentially infectious materials. Choose the appropriate glove type depending on the task. Nitrile gloves offer excellent protection against a wide range of substances, while sterile gloves are necessary for procedures requiring aseptic technique. Inspect your gloves for any tears or punctures before use; compromised gloves offer no protection. Remember that gloves should be changed frequently and disposed of properly after each use. Neglecting this simple precaution can easily lead to cross-contamination.

Gowns protect your skin and clothing from contamination. Depending on the situation, you might use disposable gowns, which are generally preferred for their ease of disposal after use. Ensure the gown properly covers your clothing and body, minimizing exposure points. Pay close attention to the proper method of fastening the gown to ensure complete coverage. When removing a gown, carefully avoid touching the outer surface to prevent the transfer of any pathogens to your clean surfaces. This is a fundamental aspect of infection control and patient safety.

Eye protection, including goggles and face shields, shields your eyes from splashes of bodily fluids or chemical exposures. Make sure that the eye protection you are using has appropriate protection against impact as well as chemical exposures, as this is often overlooked.

The fit is crucial; poorly fitting protection leaves gaps that compromise its effectiveness. Consider the potential hazards when selecting the appropriate level of eye protection. Always opt for protection that offers comprehensive coverage and a snug fit to maximize effectiveness. Relying on inadequate eye protection is a gamble you shouldn't take with your eyesight.

Respiratory protection is critical when dealing with airborne pathogens. Selecting the appropriate respirator is vital and depends heavily on the specific risk. N95 respirators, for example, filter out a significant portion of airborne particles. However, ensuring a proper seal is paramount; an improperly fitted respirator offers little protection. Furthermore, it's vital to receive proper training on how to correctly fit and use the chosen respirator. Using a respirator incorrectly renders it completely useless, leaving you vulnerable to airborne hazards. Remember, proper training and use are essential for effective protection. Neglecting either could have severe health implications.

Proper disposal of used PPE is the final and often overlooked critical step. Used PPE should be handled carefully to prevent contamination. Appropriate disposal containers and methods should always be followed meticulously, both to maintain safety and to comply with all relevant regulations. Improper disposal puts others at risk and can contribute to the spread of infection, undoing all the safety precautions you have already taken. Remember that safety is a collective responsibility. Your actions after use are as important as those during use. Therefore, a diligent, careful approach to disposal is critical to the success of any safety program.

Beyond simply knowing what PPE to use and how to use it, maintaining a heightened awareness is key. Regular training and education are necessary to stay current with best practices and adapt to new situations. Always remain informed about the appropriate PPE for specific tasks. Be proactive; seek out updated protocols and guidelines, and stay up-to-date on any new technologies or materials in PPE. Remember that even the best equipment is only as good as the person using it. Continuous learning should be part of your commitment to safety. Your own diligence plays an integral role in your safety and the safety of your colleagues.

2.3 Environmental Cleaning

Effective environmental cleaning is paramount in preventing healthcare-associated infections. It's not merely about tidying up; it's a crucial component of infection prevention and control, protecting both patients and staff. We need to remember that even seemingly minor oversights can have significant consequences. A contaminated surface can easily transmit pathogens, leading to infections that range from mild to life-threatening. This chapter will provide a practical guide to effective environmental cleaning in healthcare settings.

The first step is understanding what constitutes effective cleaning. It's not just about wiping surfaces; it's about meticulously removing visible soil and potentially infectious microorganisms. This requires using appropriate cleaning agents and techniques, ensuring thorough coverage, and paying close attention to high-touch areas—think doorknobs, light switches, bedrails, and medical equipment. Regular training for all staff is essential, to make sure everyone understands the proper methods and the importance of their role in infection control. Regular auditing of cleaning practices helps maintain high standards.

Choosing the right cleaning agents is critical. Different surfaces require different products, and using an inappropriate cleaner can damage the surface or fail to eliminate pathogens effectively. Always follow the manufacturer's instructions carefully, paying attention to dilution ratios and contact times. For example, using a solution that's too weak can fail to disinfect, whereas a solution that's too strong can damage equipment and compromise the integrity of surfaces. Many facilities now opt for environmentally friendly, low-toxicity cleaning agents to minimize the impact on the environment and staff health.

Proper disinfection protocols are equally important. Disinfection is the process of eliminating or reducing the number of pathogens on surfaces. While cleaning removes visible dirt, disinfection eliminates harmful microorganisms. This often involves using disinfectants registered with regulatory bodies to prove their effectiveness against a wide range of pathogens. It's crucial to follow the manufacturer's instructions meticulously, allowing adequate contact time for the disinfectant to work effectively, paying attention to the type of surface

being treated. In addition, we need to remember that proper ventilation is also essential to avoid inhalation of disinfectant vapors.
Cleaning schedules should be tailored to the specific environment and risk level. High-touch areas in patient rooms, for instance, require more frequent cleaning than less frequently touched surfaces in less populated areas. Establishing a robust cleaning schedule provides a structure for this vital process. In high-risk areas such as operating rooms or intensive care units, meticulous cleaning and disinfection protocols must be strictly adhered to.

Personal protective equipment (PPE) should be worn during environmental cleaning tasks. Gloves are essential to protect staff from contact with blood, body fluids, and other potentially infectious materials. Depending on the task and the environment, other PPE, such as gowns and eye protection, may also be necessary. It's very important to make sure everyone understands why PPE is important. Proper disposal of used PPE is also essential to prevent cross-contamination.

Regular monitoring and evaluation of cleaning effectiveness are vital aspects of a comprehensive environmental cleaning program. This could involve environmental culturing to assess the presence of specific pathogens or conducting audits to observe cleaning practices and adherence to protocols. These measures ensure ongoing efficacy and facilitate prompt correction of any gaps in the process. The data collected through monitoring can help identify areas needing improvement and refine cleaning protocols for optimum effectiveness and risk reduction.

Finally, a robust environmental cleaning program must be integrated into a broader infection control strategy. It should align with other infection prevention and control measures, such as hand hygiene, personal protective equipment (PPE) use, and isolation precautions. Environmental cleaning is not a standalone measure; it is an essential part of a wider strategy for minimizing the risk of infection. This collaborative approach creates a comprehensive framework to protect the health and safety of all. Remember, proactive measures—such as regular training, effective monitoring, and thorough cleaning—are not just cost-effective; they're vital for safeguarding the health of patients, visitors, and healthcare staff.

3 Medication Safety

Precisely verifying medication orders against patient records before administration is paramount. Failing to do so can lead to potentially catastrophic consequences, ranging from minor side effects to life-threatening complications. A simple discrepancy, a missed decimal point, or a wrongly interpreted abbreviation, can have devastating results, highlighting the critical need for meticulous double-checking. This practice isn't merely a guideline; it's a cornerstone of responsible and effective patient care. We must strive for absolute accuracy in every stage of the medication process.

Effective communication, both within the healthcare team and between the team and the patient, plays an undeniable role in medication safety. Open and clear dialogue ensures that everyone involved understands the medication plan thoroughly. This includes the patient's understanding of their prescribed medications, their purpose, potential side effects, and any necessary precautions. Clear and concise documentation also prevents misunderstandings and ensures continuity of care, particularly during handovers or shifts. Therefore, creating a culture of open communication fosters a safer environment for all involved.

High-alert medications demand an exceptionally high level of caution and vigilance. These are drugs with a heightened risk of causing significant patient harm if administered incorrectly. This necessitates a robust system of checks and balances, from the moment the order is written until the medication is administered. Using barcodes, double-checking dosages and routes of administration, and providing specialized training for staff administering these medications are examples of best practices. The potential for serious consequences emphasizes the need for a proactive, multi-layered approach to their handling. We must actively monitor and manage these potential dangers.

Beyond the immediate administration process, medication reconciliation is a crucial step to prevent errors. This process involves comparing a patient's medication list from various sources - previous prescriptions, home medications, and new orders - and identifying any discrepancies or potential conflicts. A comprehensive medication reconciliation at every transition point in care, such as admission, discharge, and transfers, can significantly reduce medication errors. It's not merely an administrative task; it's an integral part of ensuring patient safety. Inadequate reconciliation jeopardizes patient welfare and necessitates further scrutiny.

Adverse drug event (ADE) reporting is not only a legal requirement but a vital tool for improving patient safety. When an ADE occurs, it presents a valuable opportunity for learning and improvement.

The meticulous documentation of ADEs, along with a thorough investigation into the root cause of the error, helps identify systemic weaknesses in the medication process. This information then becomes the basis for implementing changes to prevent similar errors in the future. Transparency and a non-punitive approach to reporting are vital for fostering a culture of safety. We must encourage reporting as it aids progress.

Investing in technology to improve medication safety is crucial. Electronic medication administration records (eMARs), barcoding systems, and computerized physician order entry (CPOE) systems can significantly reduce errors related to transcription, illegible handwriting, or missed doses. These systems not only enhance accuracy but also provide real-time monitoring and tracking of medication administration. By adopting these innovative tools, we can establish a robust defense against medication errors. Moreover, regular technology updates and staff training ensure the systems function optimally and personnel remain proficient.

Finally, a culture of safety is more than just policies and procedures; it's a mindset. Open communication, teamwork, and a willingness to report errors without fear of retribution are essential components of a safe working environment. Regular training, fostering a blame-free culture, and promoting open discussion of near misses are all steps toward a more secure system of medication management. This proactive approach is the foundation of continuous improvement. We must remember that patient safety rests on the collective responsibility of every healthcare professional.

3.1 Safe Medication Practices

Proper medication handling begins with the prescription itself. Verify the order meticulously, checking for discrepancies between the physician's order, the medication administration record (MAR), and the medication label itself. Three checks are the industry standard, but remember that vigilance isn't a checklist; it's a mindset. Never rush this process; accuracy is paramount. A single missed detail can have catastrophic consequences. This is not just about following procedure, it is about safeguarding human life.

Calculating dosages accurately is another crucial step. Double-check all calculations, using independent verification whenever possible. Many facilities encourage a peer-to-peer check system precisely for this reason. Use a medication calculator if necessary; don't rely solely on mental arithmetic. Remember that even experienced professionals make mistakes, and the consequences are often severe for the patient. Errors in dosage can lead to treatment failures or adverse drug reactions. Be confident in your calculations and if you have any doubt, ask a colleague to verify.

Preparing medications demands precision and attention. The environment should be clean and well-lit. Follow all established guidelines for preparing medications, adhering strictly to the written instructions. Distractions are your enemy, so maintain focus. This is not the time for multitasking. Any deviation from the protocols can compromise patient safety. A sterile environment is crucial when dealing with injectable medications. This is not a routine task, this is about patient health.

Administration of medications requires similar caution. Always identify the patient correctly using two identifiers (e.g., name and date of birth). This seemingly simple step prevents medication errors where the wrong patient receives treatment. Before administering any medication, verify the seven rights: right patient, right medication, right dose, right route, right time, right documentation, and right reason. Never compromise on this; double-check it even when you have performed this routine many times. This is a cornerstone of patient safety.

Accurate and complete documentation is non-negotiable. Record the medication administered, the time, the route, and any relevant observations about the patient's response. Incomplete or inaccurate documentation can lead to serious complications later on. This detailed record also serves as a crucial legal and clinical record. Remember, a well-maintained record serves as a crucial audit trail. Every detail is vital in protecting the patient and your professional record.

Understanding potential adverse drug reactions is vital. Familiarize yourself with common side effects of the medications you administer. Monitor patients closely for any unexpected reactions, reporting any adverse events promptly to the appropriate authorities. Knowing the potential risks allows you to react quickly and effectively.

Knowing these potential risks will not only safeguard the patient, but will also prepare you to quickly act to handle any unexpected situations.

Staying informed on new medication guidelines and updates is an ongoing responsibility. Attend relevant continuing education programs and review updated information. The pharmaceutical landscape is constantly evolving. New research often leads to changes in medication guidelines and best practices; staying updated is crucial for safe medication practice. The goal here is to deliver the highest quality of care, and that requires ongoing learning and adaptation. Continuously updating your knowledge is crucial.

Effective communication is vital within a healthcare team. Report any medication-related concerns to your supervisor or pharmacist immediately. Don't hesitate to seek clarification if anything is unclear. Open and transparent communication reduces the likelihood of errors and ensures the best possible care for every patient. Teamwork is essential, and your questions may prevent mistakes that can have serious consequences. Your collaboration improves the overall quality of care.

Finally, remember that safe medication practices are about more than just procedures; they are about a commitment to patient well-being. Always approach your work with a mindset of attentiveness and professionalism. Patient safety is the ultimate goal. It is a continuous effort to improve our practices and maintain safety. Remember that every action has a ripple effect. Every medication you handle is a chance to prove your dedication to this duty. Every patient deserves your best attention and dedication. This commitment goes beyond following procedures; it is a profound dedication to the safety and well-being of those under your care. Safe medication practice is not merely compliance, it is a commitment to providing ethical, high-quality care.

3.2 Medication Reconciliation

Medication reconciliation is a critical process, often overlooked, yet vital for patient safety. It's the process of comparing a patient's medication list with their current medications, identifying any discrepancies, and resolving them to ensure accuracy. This seemingly simple step plays a significant role in preventing medication errors, adverse drug events, and ultimately, improving patient outcomes. Think of it as a crucial checkpoint, a vital safeguard in the complex landscape of healthcare.

Effective medication reconciliation requires a collaborative approach. It's not solely the responsibility of one individual or department; rather, it necessitates teamwork, involving physicians, nurses, pharmacists, and even the patient themselves. Open communication and the seamless exchange of information are paramount. The patient's active participation, if capable, ensures accuracy and provides valuable insight into their medication history, promoting a more personalized approach. Their involvement fosters trust and shared responsibility for their healthcare.

The process typically begins with the creation of a comprehensive medication list. This should encompass all medications the patient is currently taking, including prescription drugs, over-the-counter medications, herbal remedies, and even vitamins and supplements. Each medication should be meticulously documented, noting its name, dosage, frequency, and route of administration. Skipping even one seemingly insignificant detail can have far-reaching consequences. I've witnessed firsthand how a missed vitamin could interact dangerously with a prescribed medication.

Next comes the comparison. This critical step involves comparing the comprehensive medication list with the medications the patient is currently receiving in the new care setting - be it a hospital, nursing home, or even just a transition from one physician's care to another. Any discrepancies, whether omissions, additions, or dosage changes, must be carefully investigated and documented. This often involves verifying information with the patient, their family, or previous medical records, often uncovering significant inconsistencies that could otherwise cause complications.

Discrepancies in medication lists aren't uncommon; they can stem from poor communication between healthcare providers, incomplete patient history, or even just simple human error. The key is to systematically identify and resolve these discrepancies promptly. It's also important to understand that a discrepancy doesn't always imply an error. Sometimes, it's the result of a deliberate medication change, but the lack of communication creates a false discrepancy.

Resolving these differences requires careful consideration of the patient's medical history, current condition, and the potential interactions between medications.

Following the comparison and resolution of discrepancies, the updated medication list needs to be carefully documented and communicated to all relevant healthcare providers. This updated list serves as the definitive source of information for the patient's medication regimen, helping to prevent future errors. Accurate documentation is crucial, not just for internal consistency, but also to ensure smooth transitions of care, particularly in situations where several healthcare professionals are involved in a patient's treatment.

Beyond the direct benefits to individual patients, effective medication reconciliation contributes to broader quality improvement initiatives. By systematically identifying and addressing medication discrepancies, healthcare organizations can identify systemic issues that contribute to medication errors. This data can then be used to improve processes, implement better safeguards, and create a safer medication environment for all. It's a cyclical process of constant improvement, learning from mistakes to prevent them from happening again.

The effective implementation of medication reconciliation requires more than just a set of procedures. It necessitates a commitment to a culture of safety, where everyone involved prioritizes accurate medication administration and proactive error prevention. Regular staff training, clear protocols, and readily accessible resources are essential for creating this culture of safety. Moreover, regular audits and reviews of the process itself help ensure its effectiveness and identify any areas that require further improvement.

Furthermore, the integration of technology can significantly enhance the medication reconciliation process. Electronic health records (EHRs) can automate some aspects, reducing the potential for human error and streamlining data exchange between different healthcare providers. Smart devices and apps are also being developed to help patients actively manage their own medication lists, ensuring better patient engagement and accuracy. While technology plays a crucial role, human oversight and judgment still remain indispensable elements.

In conclusion, medication reconciliation is not merely a procedural step but a crucial safeguard in patient care. It requires a collaborative approach, meticulous attention to detail, and a dedication to a safety-conscious culture. By implementing effective medication reconciliation practices, healthcare organizations can significantly reduce medication errors, improve patient outcomes, and ultimately, contribute to a safer healthcare system for everyone. Through consistent application and continual improvement, we can make a tangible difference in the lives of countless individuals.

3.3 Adverse Drug Event Reporting

Accurate and timely reporting of adverse drug events (ADEs) is paramount for patient safety. Failure to report can lead to continued harm, hindering the development of safer practices and impacting future patient care. It's not merely a regulatory requirement; it's a moral imperative.

Understanding what constitutes an ADE is crucial. It's more than just an unexpected reaction; it encompasses any unintended, undesired, or unexpected response to a medication, occurring at therapeutic doses. This includes allergic reactions, overdoses, medication errors leading to adverse effects, and even interactions between medications, regardless of the dose. The severity can range from mild discomfort to life-threatening complications.

Reporting procedures vary depending on the healthcare setting, but the fundamental principles remain consistent. Many institutions utilize electronic reporting systems, offering a streamlined and efficient process. However, the core elements of a report are similar across all systems: accurate patient identification, details about the medication (name, dose, route, frequency), a clear description of the event, its severity, the outcome, and any interventions undertaken. Supporting documentation, such as lab results, is often invaluable.

Thorough documentation is your first line of defense. Clearly record the details of the ADE within the patient's medical record. This ensures a complete picture of the event, allowing for better analysis and future prevention efforts. Remember, meticulous documentation is not just about complying with regulations; it's about protecting your patient and contributing to broader safety improvements within your healthcare facility. Take the time, be precise, and make sure everything is clear. Don't leave anything out; every detail is crucial in understanding the entire context.

Investigating ADEs is more than simply filing a report. It requires a systematic approach, often involving a multidisciplinary team. This team, depending on the severity of the event, may include nurses, pharmacists, physicians, and risk managers. The goal is not to assign blame but to identify contributing factors and system-wide issues that contributed to the ADE. A thorough root cause analysis can unearth systemic weaknesses in medication ordering, dispensing, administration, or monitoring processes.

The information gathered from ADE reports feeds into larger databases. These databases, both national and international, play a crucial role in pharmacovigilance. The data collected allows for trends to be identified, helping researchers and regulatory agencies assess the safety profiles of medications and prompt timely interventions, such as warnings or drug recalls. Your contribution, no matter how seemingly small, contributes to a global effort to improve patient safety. You're not just reporting an event; you're participating in a wider safety net.

Preventing future ADEs requires a proactive, multi-faceted approach. This involves regular staff training on medication administration, effective communication amongst healthcare professionals, robust medication reconciliation protocols, and the use of technological advancements like barcoding systems and computerized physician order entry. Implementing and enforcing these measures helps create a culture of safety where everyone shares the responsibility for preventing ADEs.

Beyond formal reporting systems, there's the human aspect of ADE reporting. If you witness or suspect an ADE, report it immediately. This includes near-misses; near misses, or potential ADEs that are caught before harm occurs, are equally important in preventing future events. The information gained from these near misses is crucial in identifying potential vulnerabilities in systems and prevents future occurrences. Do not hesitate to report, even if you are unsure, it's better to be cautious and inform your superiors rather than to let a critical matter pass unreported. Remember, your actions can directly impact the safety and well-being of your patients. This extends to supporting your colleagues, fostering an environment where reporting is not only accepted but actively encouraged.

Finally, remember that ADE reporting is not about pointing fingers. It's a collaborative process aiming to improve patient safety. By contributing to this process, you play a vital role in protecting your patients and shaping a safer healthcare environment for everyone. It's a team effort, a shared responsibility; by working together, by sharing knowledge, by openly reporting any adverse event, regardless of the reason, we contribute to a safer environment for everyone. Every report brings us closer to a future where such events are minimised, a future where the overall safety of patients is guaranteed.

3.4 High-Alert Medications

High-alert medications demand heightened vigilance due to their potential for significant harm if administered incorrectly. These medications, often affecting critical bodily functions, require meticulous attention to detail at every stage - from ordering and dispensing to administration and documentation. Errors involving these drugs can have devastating consequences, ranging from serious adverse events to patient fatalities. Therefore, robust safety protocols are crucial.

A multi-pronged approach is necessary to minimize the risks associated with high-alert medications. First, a comprehensive understanding of each medication's properties, including its mechanism of action, potential side effects, and contraindications, is paramount. Healthcare professionals must remain updated on the latest research and guidelines, continuously refining their knowledge base. This ongoing education ensures a deeper understanding of each medication's intricacies. Regular training programs, supplemented by easily accessible resources like updated formularies and online databases, can greatly contribute to the proficiency of staff handling high-alert drugs.

Strict adherence to established procedures is another cornerstone of safe handling. Double-checking orders, verifying patient identification, and utilizing independent double-checks, especially when administering parenteral medications, are not mere formalities; they are essential safeguards. Standardized procedures, consistently followed, dramatically minimize the potential for human error. Every step of the medication administration process should include verification measures, with clear documentation at each point to create a robust audit trail. Discrepancies should trigger immediate investigation, allowing for corrective action.

Technology plays an increasingly important role in enhancing the safety of high-alert medication management. Automated dispensing cabinets, barcode scanning, and electronic health records (EHRs) can significantly reduce errors associated with transcription, dispensing, and administration. These systems provide real-time monitoring, alerting staff to potential discrepancies and inconsistencies before they lead to serious incidents. Regular maintenance and staff training on the utilization of these technological tools are crucial to their effective operation. These preventative measures are integral components in medication safety procedures.

The creation of a strong safety culture, however, transcends checklists and technologies. It necessitates open communication, where staff feel empowered to report errors or near misses without fear of retribution. A culture of transparency allows for identification of systemic weaknesses, fostering a proactive approach to risk mitigation. This collaborative environment creates a setting in which staff members feel comfortable sharing experiences and knowledge to achieve greater safety and a commitment to shared responsibility. Regular safety huddles and debriefings provide avenues for collective problem-solving, streamlining processes, and continually

improving safety protocols.
Effective communication is also crucial during the entire medication administration process. Accurate and complete documentation is essential for maintaining a comprehensive patient record and aids in any potential investigation or review of the medication administration process. Clear and concise communication between healthcare providers, including during medication rounds and handoffs, is critical to ensuring consistent and safe medication practices. It's essential to establish a system that allows for seamless transfer of information to reduce errors and potential omissions during medication changes or transitions of care. Employing a system of verification and double-checking with collaborative communication can help ensure the accuracy of medication orders.
Finally, post-event analysis is not merely an administrative chore; it is a vital learning opportunity. Thorough investigation into medication errors, regardless of severity, can highlight deficiencies in existing processes and policies, enabling corrective actions to prevent recurrence. Regular audits of medication administration records are not just regulatory requirements, but are invaluable tools for identifying trends, revealing underlying issues, and continually refining safety protocols. This continuous improvement approach ensures the constant refinement of protocols, reinforcing the commitment to patient safety. Adopting these strategies results in a safer healthcare environment.

3.5 Medication Errors Prevention

Proper medication administration is paramount. Double-checking medication orders against patient charts, meticulously verifying dosages, and carefully administering medications using the six rights (right patient, right medication, right dose, right route, right time, right documentation) are not just guidelines; they're lifelines. Failing to adhere to these principles can lead to devastating consequences, highlighting the critical need for unwavering vigilance. Every single medication interaction, from the initial order to the final documentation, demands meticulous attention to detail. Remember that even a seemingly minor oversight can have significant repercussions.

A comprehensive understanding of the medications themselves is just as vital. Knowing potential drug interactions, side effects, and contraindications is crucial. Regularly updating knowledge through continuing education and actively utilizing available resources such as drug formularies and clinical guidelines is essential for every healthcare professional. This continuous learning fosters a proactive approach, mitigating risks and improving patient outcomes. One should consider attending relevant professional development courses and workshops. These enhance familiarity with new drugs and updated guidelines.

Teamwork is undeniably crucial in medication error prevention. Open communication, collaborative decision-making, and mutual respect among healthcare professionals contribute to a robust safety net. Regular interdisciplinary rounds and structured communication protocols promote proactive identification and resolution of potential medication safety concerns. A collaborative environment cultivates a culture of shared responsibility for patient safety, minimizing the likelihood of errors. This collaborative approach fosters a safe environment where individuals are comfortable voicing concerns.

Effective use of technology can significantly enhance medication safety. Barcoding systems, automated dispensing cabinets, and electronic medication administration records (eMARs) are examples of how technology aids in reducing errors. These technological aids provide real-time medication tracking, promoting accuracy and minimizing the potential for human error. The implementation of these systems, however, requires appropriate training and ongoing monitoring to maximize their effectiveness and integration into existing workflows. Technological advancement is a powerful tool, but its implementation requires both proper planning and effective staff training.

The establishment of robust reporting systems is fundamental. A transparent and non-punitive environment for reporting medication errors is essential for learning and improvement. Analyzing reported errors, identifying patterns, and implementing corrective actions are all part of a continuous quality improvement cycle. This continuous process enhances safety, leading to safer medication practices across the healthcare system. A system for reporting errors should be designed to encourage open communication without fear of reprisal. A blame-free environment is essential for creating a safe learning environment.

Patient education plays a significant, albeit often overlooked, role. Empowering patients to actively participate in their medication management by understanding their medications, potential side effects, and the importance of adherence is crucial. Open communication with patients fosters a partnership in their care, contributing to the overall safety and effectiveness of their medication regimen. Understanding their medications helps patients understand what to report. This contributes to the early detection of adverse drug reactions. Patient involvement fosters safety and improves outcomes. Finally, remember the human element. Fatigue, stress, and distractions can significantly impact performance and increase the risk of errors. Implementing strategies to mitigate these factors, such as adequate staffing levels, appropriate breaks, and promoting a supportive work environment, significantly reduces the likelihood of medication errors. Supporting healthcare professionals is essential to ensuring the delivery of quality and safe care. This involves prioritizing their well-being, as stressed professionals can more easily fall prey to mistakes. Professional well-being directly correlates with patient safety.

4 Patient Safety Initiatives

Implementing effective fall prevention strategies is paramount to patient safety. A comprehensive approach requires a multidisciplinary team, including nurses, physicians, physical therapists, and even housekeeping staff. Regular risk assessments, tailored to each patient's individual needs and mobility limitations, are crucial. These assessments should consider factors such as age, medical history, medication side effects, and the environment. For example, a patient with a history of falls or on multiple medications that could cause dizziness would require more frequent checks and potentially assistive devices. Simple changes, such as ensuring adequate lighting and removing clutter from pathways, can significantly reduce fall risks.

Beyond the assessment, implementing preventative measures is essential. Bed alarms, appropriately used, can alert staff to a patient attempting to get out of bed unassisted. However, overuse can lead to alarm fatigue, diminishing their effectiveness. Proper training for staff on the correct application and use of assistive devices, such as walkers and canes, is key. This includes ensuring patients understand and are comfortable using them. Non-slip socks, strategically placed grab bars, and raised toilet seats are examples of simple yet highly effective interventions. Regular mobility assessments, perhaps daily, can identify subtle changes in a patient's gait or balance. Early identification allows for timely adjustments and minimizes the likelihood of a fall.

Pressure ulcer prevention requires diligent attention to detail and a proactive approach. The cornerstone of prevention lies in meticulous skin assessment. Nurses should regularly inspect the patient's skin, paying close attention to bony prominences. Any redness, warmth, or changes in skin integrity warrant immediate attention. Regular repositioning of bedridden patients is critical, typically every two hours or more frequently, depending on the patient's condition and risk factors. This alleviates pressure on specific areas, improving circulation. Special mattresses and cushions, designed to redistribute pressure and reduce friction, should be employed when deemed necessary. Maintaining optimal nutrition and hydration is also fundamental, as proper nutrition promotes healthy skin and aids in wound healing. Nutritional consultations can help address any dietary deficiencies, optimizing the patient's overall health.

Skin care is another key element. Keeping the skin clean and dry is essential. Using moisturizers can prevent dryness and cracking, increasing the skin's resistance to breakdown. Gentle cleansing, avoiding harsh soaps and excessive friction, is crucial. It's essential for healthcare providers to understand the underlying pathophysiology of pressure ulcers, which involves prolonged pressure disrupting blood flow to tissues. The knowledge allows them to implement evidence-based prevention strategies, rather than relying on intuition or outdated practices. Regular education for staff and the implementation of standardized protocols will improve consistency in care and reduce the incidence of pressure ulcers.

Beyond individual patient care, a strong organizational commitment to patient safety is vital. This includes establishing clear protocols for fall and pressure ulcer prevention, providing ongoing staff education and training, actively monitoring outcomes, and fostering a culture of safety reporting. The organization should regularly review and update their policies to incorporate the latest evidence-based practices. This iterative process of improvement involves analyzing the data collected from incidents, identifying any patterns or contributing factors, and implementing changes to prevent similar incidents from happening again. For instance, if a particular type of medication is identified as a risk factor for falls, the organization may review its medication prescribing guidelines. Open communication between staff members, patients, and families is crucial, fostering a cooperative environment that prioritizes safety and allows for proactive risk management. A strong reporting system without penalizing staff for reporting near misses or adverse events will allow for transparent learning and improvements to patient care. Ultimately, patient safety initiatives are not just about following protocols but about fostering a culture of care where safety is a shared responsibility.

4.1 Fall Prevention Strategies

Falls are a significant concern in healthcare settings, leading to injuries, extended hospital stays, and increased healthcare costs. Implementing a comprehensive fall prevention program is paramount. This requires a multi-faceted approach involving risk assessment, environmental modifications, and staff education. A proactive strategy minimizes risk and fosters a safer environment for patients.

Effective fall risk assessment is crucial. It's not just about age; it involves a thorough evaluation of each patient's individual factors. Consider their medical history, medications, cognitive status, mobility limitations, and visual acuity. Use validated assessment tools, regularly reassessing patients' risk levels, especially after significant changes in their condition or medication regimen. Documenting these assessments meticulously is vital for tracking progress and demonstrating adherence to best practices. Remember, consistency is key; consistent assessments and documentation are crucial for improved patient safety and outcomes.

Environmental modifications play a significant role. Consider the patient's room layout. Ensure clear pathways, adequate lighting, and removal of clutter. Non-slip mats in bathrooms and bedside areas are essential. Bedside rails should be appropriately used and maintained. Regular safety checks of the patient's environment are mandatory. Furthermore, the hospital or healthcare facility should regularly evaluate the overall environment to identify and rectify potential fall hazards proactively. This is where a team effort really shines; collaboration with housekeeping and maintenance teams ensures consistent safety protocols across the entire facility.

Staff education is crucial. All healthcare personnel should receive regular training on fall prevention techniques. This includes understanding fall risk factors, proper use of assistive devices, and safe patient handling procedures. Furthermore, staff must be empowered to report near misses and falls promptly, allowing for immediate corrective actions and a thorough investigation. This should be reinforced through regular in-services, continuing education opportunities, and open communication channels. Training shouldn't be a one-time event; it's an ongoing process to maintain and refine knowledge and skills.

Assistive devices are vital. Properly fitting and utilizing assistive devices like walkers, canes, and wheelchairs are critical. Staff must be trained to correctly fit these devices, assess patient comfort, and ensure appropriate usage. Regular maintenance and inspection of these devices are also crucial. Furthermore, providing patients and their families with education on safe device use is an important aspect of this strategy. The right assistive device can significantly reduce fall risk, provided it's used correctly and consistently. Remember, the patient's comfort and safety should always be paramount.

Medication management is another critical component. Regularly review patients' medications, paying close attention to those with known side effects like dizziness or drowsiness. Work collaboratively with pharmacists to optimize medication regimens, minimizing the risk of adverse reactions that may increase fall propensity. Promptly address any medication-related concerns, consulting with physicians as needed. Detailed medication reconciliation ensures accuracy and avoids potential conflicts. The safety of our patients depends upon attention to these details.

Finally, consider the broader systems of care. Establish clear protocols for responding to falls, ensuring prompt assessment and treatment. Analyze fall data to identify trends and implement targeted interventions. Continuous quality improvement measures are crucial. Regular review of the fall prevention program helps us identify areas for improvement and adapt to changing circumstances. A culture of safety, emphasizing proactive risk management, is essential to create a fall-free environment. This requires commitment from every member of the healthcare team.

4.2 Pressure Ulcer Prevention

Regular repositioning is key; it's not just about turning a patient; it's about preventing prolonged pressure on any one area. Think of it like this: imagine holding a heavy book in one hand for hours. Your hand would ache, right? The same principle applies to a patient's skin. Frequent changes in position redistribute pressure, allowing blood flow to reach all areas, preventing tissue damage. Aim for repositioning at least every two hours, but more frequently if needed, especially for patients with limited mobility or existing pressure injuries. Use a structured schedule, documenting each repositioning to maintain consistency.

Maintaining optimal nutrition is also vital. Proper nutrition provides the body with the essential building blocks for tissue repair and growth, which is crucial for wound healing and pressure ulcer prevention. Malnutrition weakens the skin, making it more susceptible to breakdown. Encourage patients to eat a balanced diet rich in protein, vitamins, and minerals. Collaborate with dieticians for personalized nutritional plans to ensure patients receive adequate nutrition, addressing any deficiencies promptly. Monitor their food intake and weight regularly to track progress and make adjustments as necessary. For patients with swallowing difficulties or poor appetites, consider nutritional supplements under medical supervision.

Skin assessment is fundamental. Regular inspections are the cornerstone of pressure ulcer prevention. Each assessment needs to be thorough, examining the entire body for any signs of redness, warmth, swelling, or changes in skin texture or sensation. Pay particular attention to areas prone to pressure, such as heels, ankles, hips, and sacrum. Use standardized tools to document findings; a simple photograph can be invaluable. Remember, early detection is crucial; promptly address any skin changes to prevent ulcer development. Document everything meticulously, recording the location, size, and any other relevant details. Your thorough record-keeping is critical for tracking progress and informing future care plans.

Proper support surfaces are essential. They distribute weight evenly, reducing pressure points and decreasing the risk of pressure ulcers. There's a range of surfaces available, from simple foam mattresses to advanced air-fluidized beds. The choice of support surface should be tailored to the patient's individual needs and risk assessment. Remember to regularly check the condition of the support surface, ensuring it remains clean, undamaged, and provides adequate support. For patients at high risk, consider consulting with a wound care specialist to determine the most appropriate support surface to prevent pressure ulcers and promote optimal healing. Using the right surface alone will not prevent ulcers entirely, it needs to be used in conjunction with other preventive methods.

Maintaining skin hygiene is surprisingly important. Clean, dry skin is less prone to breakdown. Regularly cleanse the skin with mild soap and water, avoiding harsh chemicals or excessive friction. Use a gentle moisturizing lotion to keep the skin hydrated and supple. Pay close attention to areas prone to moisture, such as underarms, groin, and buttocks, keeping them dry and using absorbent products as needed. Remember, skin moisture from perspiration, incontinence, or wound exudates creates the perfect environment for bacterial growth and skin breakdown. Proper hygiene reduces the risk of infection and aids in preventing pressure ulcers.

Patient and family education is crucial. Empowering patients and their families to actively participate in pressure ulcer prevention significantly improves outcomes. Explain the importance of regular repositioning, the role of nutrition in maintaining skin integrity, and the significance of reporting any skin changes promptly. Provide clear instructions on how to perform skin care correctly and identify potential risks. Encourage active participation in the care plan and address any concerns or questions. Remember to use simple language and visual aids to improve understanding.

Finally, consider the overall clinical picture. Underlying medical conditions such as diabetes, poor circulation, and incontinence greatly increase the risk of pressure ulcers. Work closely with the patient's healthcare team to address these conditions aggressively. By optimizing blood sugar control, managing circulation issues, and implementing effective incontinence management strategies, we can significantly reduce the patient's vulnerability to pressure ulcers. This holistic approach is essential for achieving the best possible outcomes, ensuring the patient's comfort, and preventing potentially devastating complications.

5 Emergency Preparedness

Developing a comprehensive emergency plan is crucial for any healthcare facility. It's not simply about having a plan on paper; it's about regular drills, staff training, and a commitment to continuous improvement. This ensures everyone understands their roles and responsibilities during a crisis. Failure to adequately prepare can lead to chaos, increased patient harm, and significant legal repercussions. Proactive measures, like regular testing of emergency power systems and communication networks, are indispensable.

Effective communication is the lifeblood of any emergency response. Your plan should clearly define communication channels and protocols, ensuring that information flows swiftly and accurately among staff, patients, and external agencies like emergency medical services. Designate specific individuals as communication leads to avoid confusion and delays. Consider using various communication tools - pagers, text alerts, and even a public address system - depending on the nature of the event. Regular training in the use of these systems is paramount, mimicking real-life scenarios to build confidence and competence. Don't forget to regularly update contact information for all staff and external stakeholders.

Disaster planning must include various scenarios, extending beyond routine power outages to encompass major events like natural disasters, pandemics, and acts of terrorism. Consider geographic location and vulnerability to specific hazards when developing your plans. Your plan should address evacuation procedures, including the safe transportation of patients with varying levels of mobility. Establish clear meeting points both inside and outside the facility and provide detailed instructions on how to reach them safely. Having designated areas for shelter and providing essential supplies like water, food, and medical equipment is essential for extended emergencies. Remember, the more comprehensive the scenarios your team plans for, the more likely they'll be prepared for unexpected emergencies.

A robust code response system is essential for handling medical emergencies within the facility. Each code (e.g., Code Blue for cardiac arrest, Code Red for fire) should trigger a specific set of actions. These actions should be clearly defined, practiced during drills, and easily accessible to all staff members. Ensure all team members know the location of emergency equipment, including defibrillators, oxygen tanks, and first-aid supplies. Clear signage and easy navigation are key. The goal is to react swiftly and efficiently, minimizing response times and preventing further harm. Consistent training and regular review of the system is essential.

Emergency preparedness involves much more than just having a plan. It's about fostering a culture of safety and preparedness within your organization. This involves staff training, regular drills, and continuous evaluation of the plan's effectiveness. It's about ensuring that every member of the team understands their responsibilities and is confident in their ability to respond effectively. Regular drills should simulate different types of emergencies, testing the plan's effectiveness and identifying any weaknesses. This process needs to be regularly documented and reviewed. Post-drill analysis allows for improvement and refinements in the emergency response system.

Finally, remember that emergency preparedness is a continuous process, not a one-time event. Regularly review and update your emergency plan, incorporating lessons learned from drills and actual emergencies. Changes in staff, technology, or regulations may necessitate updates. Stay informed about emerging threats and hazards relevant to your area. Collaboration with local emergency services is also vital, ensuring seamless coordination during a crisis. Remember, preparedness is not just about preventing disasters; it's about mitigating their impact and ensuring the safety of your patients and staff. The aim is to transform your organization from reacting to emergencies to proactively anticipating and mitigating risks, fostering confidence in your ability to handle any unforeseen challenge.

5.1 Disaster Planning

Effective disaster planning is crucial for maintaining the safety and continuity of healthcare services. It's not merely a checklist; it's a dynamic, evolving process requiring continuous review and adaptation based on evolving threats and lessons learned. We must move beyond simple emergency response protocols to a holistic approach that anticipates various scenarios, mitigates risks proactively, and ensures a swift, coordinated response when disaster strikes.

A robust plan incorporates detailed risk assessments. Consider geographical vulnerabilities - are you prone to earthquakes, floods, hurricanes, or wildfires? What are the potential impacts on your facility, staff, and patients? Inventory your resources; assess the resilience of your infrastructure, including power, water, and communication systems. Identifying weaknesses allows for targeted mitigation efforts, such as investing in backup generators or establishing alternative communication channels. These aren't just hypothetical questions; they are essential steps in building a resilient healthcare system.

Staff training is paramount. Regular drills and simulations, mirroring real-life scenarios, ensure everyone understands their roles and responsibilities. This extends beyond clinicians; administrative staff, maintenance personnel, and security guards all play a vital part in a coordinated emergency response. Clear communication protocols are essential. Designate roles for incident command, ensuring clear lines of authority and accountability. Practice using communication systems - radios, pagers, mobile phones - to ensure seamless information flow during an emergency. Don't assume technology will always work; have backup plans, and practice those too.

Patient evacuation procedures must be meticulously planned and regularly practiced. This includes establishing clear routes, designating safe zones, and identifying transport options. Consider patients with diverse needs, including those requiring oxygen, dialysis, or other specialized care. Their specific requirements must be factored into the evacuation plan. Furthermore, maintaining a comprehensive inventory of medical supplies and equipment is critical. This inventory should detail storage locations, quantities, and expiry dates. Regular checks and replenishments are crucial, preventing shortages during emergencies.

The plan should account for potential disruptions to external support systems. This includes establishing relationships with neighboring hospitals, establishing agreements for mutual aid, and identifying alternative supply chains. Collaboration is key, as a single hospital cannot solve every problem. Building a network of supporting organizations enhances resilience. Consider your community. Understanding your community's vulnerabilities and the potential consequences of a disaster on your patients' families allows you to develop a response that supports both patients and the community as a whole.

Communication with the public is just as essential. Develop strategies for informing the public about the emergency and providing updates. Consider multiple communication channels - websites, social media, local news outlets. Clear, consistent messaging fosters trust and prevents panic. Regularly review and update your disaster plan. The healthcare landscape is constantly changing, as are the potential threats. Conduct regular reviews, incorporating lessons learned from past incidents or drills. This is an ongoing process, not a one-time event.

Post-disaster recovery plans are just as important as the initial response. They outline the procedures for resuming normal operations, assessing damages, and providing continued care. This should include a detailed plan for restoring infrastructure, replenishing supplies, and addressing the mental health needs of both staff and patients. Consider the psychological impact of a disaster. Stress and trauma are real possibilities for those who were directly involved. Plan for psychological first aid and access to mental health support. This will aid in long-term recovery, ensuring everyone involved can begin to rebuild their lives. Disaster planning isn't just about safety; it is about building a resilient healthcare system capable of enduring the unexpected and emerging stronger than ever.

5.2 Code Response Protocols

Effective code response protocols are crucial for maintaining a safe and efficient healthcare environment. A well-defined protocol ensures a swift, coordinated response to critical situations, minimizing harm to patients and staff. This involves clear communication channels, designated roles, and pre-established procedures, tailored to the specific needs of the healthcare facility. Regular drills and simulations are vital for ensuring staff proficiency and team cohesion during emergencies.

Understanding the specific codes used within your facility is paramount. These codes, often color-coded or numerically designated, signal the nature of the emergency—from cardiac arrest to fire or a hazardous materials spill. Familiarization with these codes is essential for every member of the healthcare team, regardless of their specific role. This includes nurses, doctors, support staff, and even volunteers. Effective training programs are indispensable for ensuring everyone can respond appropriately and effectively.

Clear communication is the cornerstone of a successful code response. Designated communication channels, such as dedicated phones or paging systems, must be readily available and in perfect working order. During a code, communication should be concise and unambiguous, using standardized terminology to avoid confusion and ensure everyone understands the situation. This includes relaying essential information such as the patient's location, the nature of the emergency, and the resources required. The designated leader should clearly articulate the plan, ensuring everyone understands their role.

The success of any code response relies heavily on team dynamics and pre-assigned roles. Each team member should have a defined role and responsibility. For example, one person may be responsible for initiating the code, another for providing basic life support, and others for managing equipment and facilitating communication. This hierarchical structure streamlines the response process, ensuring efficiency and minimizing confusion in the midst of a stressful emergency. Regular team drills are important to ensure all staff are trained effectively and understand these roles.

Post-code debriefings are critical for continuous improvement. These debriefings provide a platform to analyze the response, identify areas for improvement, and implement corrective actions. This systematic approach ensures that the healthcare team learns from each incident, refining its processes to enhance efficiency and effectiveness in subsequent emergencies. It's essential to create a culture of constructive feedback, encouraging open communication and a willingness to identify mistakes without blame. Focus should be on preventative measures that prevent recurrences.

Equipment readiness is another essential element. All necessary equipment, including defibrillators, emergency medications, and airway management devices, must be readily accessible and meticulously maintained. Regular inspections and maintenance schedules are necessary to guarantee the functionality of the equipment, preventing delays or malfunctions during a critical response. Knowing the precise location and functionality of every piece of equipment is a prerequisite for efficiency.

Finally, preparedness extends beyond immediate responses. Having robust disaster plans encompassing all conceivable scenarios is critical. These plans should integrate various emergency responses and should detail procedures for evacuation, securing patient records, and maintaining communication with external agencies. Regular reviews and updates to these plans are essential for adapting to changing needs and evolving best practices. Preparing for the unexpected ensures that the healthcare facility can handle all situations safely and effectively. This is vital for the safety of both staff and patients.

5.3 Emergency Communication

Effective emergency communication is the cornerstone of a successful response to any healthcare crisis. It's not just about having the right technology; it's about having a well-rehearsed, multifaceted system that ensures everyone receives vital information quickly and accurately. A breakdown in communication can lead to delays in treatment, misallocation of resources, and even preventable deaths. Therefore, robust protocols are not merely advisable, but essential. Clear and concise communication during emergencies relies heavily on pre-established protocols. These shouldn't be static documents gathering dust on a shelf; they should be regularly reviewed, updated, and practiced. Drills and simulations are vital. These exercises allow staff to familiarize themselves with the system, identify weaknesses, and refine procedures. Think of it like a fire drill; the familiarity reduces panic and improves the overall response. Regular training is not merely a suggestion; it's a non-negotiable part of ensuring effective emergency communication. Your life, and the lives of those in your care, may depend on it.

Beyond drills, your communication strategy must consider multiple channels. Relying solely on one method, such as internal paging systems, is risky. What happens if the system fails? A diverse approach incorporates various communication tools, including pagers, text messages, emails, and even a public address system. Redundancy is critical; this ensures a message can reach its intended recipients regardless of technical glitches or overwhelming demand. Consider the accessibility of each method; some staff might not always have access to email, for example, which necessitates the inclusion of alternative channels. This is not just about efficiency; it's about resilience.

Effective communication also requires clear roles and responsibilities. Each team member needs a defined role within the emergency response plan, with clear communication pathways. Knowing who is responsible for notifying specific individuals, updating dashboards, or coordinating external agencies ensures a streamlined process and prevents confusion. Having a designated spokesperson to communicate with the media or the public helps manage external perceptions and ensures a unified message. This avoids conflicting reports and maintains public trust and transparency. Without a clear chain of command, even the best-laid plans can unravel swiftly.

The language used during an emergency must be precise and unambiguous. Avoid jargon and technical terms that might confuse those unfamiliar with medical terminology. Use plain language, and be sure the message is easy to understand under pressure. Consider different communication needs. Visual aids, such as simple diagrams or color-coded maps, can supplement verbal instructions, particularly for those who may have difficulty understanding complex instructions. This is not just about understanding; it's about ensuring that every member of your team is empowered to act swiftly.

Finally, post-incident debriefing is as important as the emergency response itself. This provides an opportunity to identify areas for improvement. What worked well? What could have been improved? Were there communication breakdowns? This review is crucial for refining your communication plan and strengthening your overall preparedness. The goal isn't to assign blame, but to learn from both successes and failures. This is not merely a matter of compliance. It's about a continuous cycle of refinement. A commitment to learning from each response will inevitably lead to a safer environment for everyone. By consistently analyzing and refining your communication protocol, you build a resilient and effective system, transforming your emergency response from a reactive measure into a proactive safeguard. This consistent improvement ensures that future emergencies are met not with uncertainty, but with well-honed competence.

6 Quality Improvement in Healthcare

Effective quality improvement hinges on a systematic approach. Start by clearly defining your goals. What specific aspects of healthcare safety are you aiming to enhance? Are you targeting medication errors, infection rates, or perhaps fall incidents? Precisely outlining objectives ensures focus and allows for measurable progress. Remember, vague aims lead to vague results; a sharply defined goal provides a concrete target to strive for. This clarity also aids in selecting the appropriate quality improvement methodology.

Data is the bedrock of any successful quality improvement initiative. You need reliable, comprehensive data to pinpoint areas needing attention. This involves more than just collecting numbers; it necessitates selecting relevant metrics, establishing consistent data collection methods, and ensuring data accuracy and completeness. Think about patient falls: Simply tracking the number of falls is insufficient; you'll need to analyze the circumstances of each fall, identify contributing factors like medication side effects or environmental hazards, and then correlate this data with patient characteristics. Only then can effective interventions be designed. This detailed, multi-faceted approach to data analysis is crucial for identifying the root causes of problems, and not just addressing surface-level symptoms.

Once you've gathered and analyzed your data, the next step is identifying the root cause of the problem. This isn't simply about finding the immediate cause; it's about digging deeper to uncover the underlying systemic issues. The "five whys" technique, a simple yet powerful tool, can be invaluable here. By repeatedly asking "why" until you reach the fundamental cause, you unveil the systemic factors contributing to the problem. For example, if many medication errors stem from illegible handwriting on medication orders, the immediate cause is poor handwriting, but the root cause might be a lack of electronic prescribing systems, insufficient staff training on legible writing, or even a culture that doesn't prioritize clear communication. Addressing the root cause, not just the symptoms, is essential for sustainable improvement.

Continuous quality improvement is a journey, not a destination. It's an ongoing process of monitoring, evaluating, and refining your approach. Regular review of your data, reassessment of your goals, and a willingness to adapt your strategies are critical for sustained success. Implementing changes in small, manageable steps minimizes disruption and allows for continuous monitoring and adjustment, enabling early identification of any unintended consequences. Furthermore, engaging all staff members, from doctors and nurses to administrative personnel, ensures a team-based, collective approach that facilitates both buy-in and long-term success. This collaborative process, fueled by regular feedback loops, is what turns improvement into a cultural norm.

Cultivating a robust safety culture is paramount. This involves creating an environment where reporting errors is not viewed as blameworthy, but as an opportunity for learning and improvement. Open communication channels, a culture of trust, and constructive feedback mechanisms are essential for fostering this environment. Establish clear reporting systems, ensure confidentiality, and demonstrate visible commitment from leadership to create an atmosphere where reporting is not only encouraged but valued. Remember, a blame-free culture empowers healthcare professionals to openly identify and address safety concerns, ultimately leading to a safer and more effective healthcare system. It's about fostering a collective responsibility for patient safety, shifting from individual accountability to shared responsibility and a commitment to continuous learning. This fosters a more resilient and adaptable healthcare system, better equipped to handle future challenges.

6.1 Data Collection & Analysis

Effective data collection is the cornerstone of any successful quality improvement initiative. Without accurate, reliable data, improvements are guesswork, potentially leading to wasted resources and, critically, continued patient harm. We must meticulously plan data collection to ensure its relevance to our objectives. This involves clearly defining the specific safety issue we're addressing—for instance, medication errors related to high-alert medications—and identifying the key data points needed to understand its prevalence and contributing factors. Careful consideration of data sources is also crucial; these might include incident reports, electronic health records, medication administration records, and even direct observation of healthcare practices. Remember, poorly chosen metrics lead to misleading conclusions.

A well-designed data collection tool is essential. It should be user-friendly, minimizing the time healthcare professionals need to complete it and thus maximizing participation. Ambiguity must be eliminated, using clear, concise questions with pre-defined response options wherever possible. This ensures consistency and minimizes variability in data interpretation. For example, a checklist for hand hygiene compliance is preferable to an open-ended question about handwashing frequency. Data entry should be streamlined, ideally integrating directly with existing electronic systems. This automation minimizes the risk of data entry errors and facilitates analysis.

Data analysis moves beyond simple descriptive statistics. We need to identify trends, patterns, and relationships within the collected data. This might involve calculating rates of specific incidents, analyzing correlations between different variables, and visualizing data using charts and graphs to communicate findings effectively. For instance, tracking the number of medication errors per month may reveal a seasonal trend, offering potential insights into contributing factors. Sophisticated statistical methods, such as regression analysis, can uncover more subtle relationships between variables, providing a deeper understanding of the root causes of safety issues.

Visualizing the data is not just about aesthetics; it's a powerful communication tool. Clear, concise visualizations, such as bar charts, line graphs, and pie charts, make complex data readily understandable for healthcare professionals across various disciplines. These visualizations help to highlight trends and patterns, facilitating effective communication with colleagues and decision-makers. Consider your audience when choosing a visualization method - a simple bar chart is often more effective than a complex scatter plot when communicating results to a non-statistical audience. Interactive dashboards can allow exploration of the data, enabling a more in-depth understanding.

Finally, the interpretation of the data must be evidence-based and objective. Avoid subjective interpretations or drawing conclusions unsupported by the data. Always consider possible biases or limitations within the data collection process. For instance, underreporting of incidents is a common problem, and we need to account for this when analyzing results. Once the analysis is complete, the findings must be disseminated effectively to the relevant stakeholders, including clinicians, administrators, and quality improvement teams. Recommendations for improvement, based on the evidence, should then be implemented, monitored, and evaluated to ensure lasting positive change. Transparency and collaboration are crucial in this process to build a safety culture and foster continuous improvement. Effective data analysis is not an endpoint; it's an ongoing cycle of learning, improvement, and further refinement.

6.2 Performance Improvement

Effective performance improvement hinges on a systematic approach, not a haphazard collection of fixes. Start by clearly defining your goals. What specific areas need improvement? Are you aiming to reduce medication errors, decrease patient falls, or improve hand hygiene compliance? Setting measurable, achievable, relevant, and time-bound (SMART) goals provides a concrete roadmap. Without clearly defined objectives, your efforts will lack focus and direction, hindering progress. Remember that success is measured not just by ambition, but by tangible results.

Data is your most valuable tool. Comprehensive data collection is essential; it's the foundation upon which you build your strategy. Carefully examine existing data sources. Look at incident reports, near misses, patient satisfaction surveys, and infection control data. These sources offer invaluable insights into areas needing attention. Don't be afraid to delve into the details - patterns may not be immediately obvious, but persistent investigation frequently uncovers hidden connections and trends pointing towards the root causes of your performance issues. Remember that quality data ensures accurate problem identification and the development of robust solutions. Once data analysis reveals performance gaps, investigate the root causes. A surface-level fix might seem convenient, but it risks masking the underlying problem, leading to recurrence. Employ root cause analysis techniques such as the "5 Whys" method. Probing beyond immediate explanations uncovers the systemic issues hindering optimal performance. This deeper understanding informs more effective and sustainable solutions. Don't just treat the symptoms; resolve the underlying issues driving poor performance to create lasting change.

Develop and implement corrective actions. Once you've identified the root causes, design specific, targeted interventions. This may involve revising protocols, providing additional training, or acquiring new equipment. Involve staff in the process; their input is essential for buy-in and successful implementation. Remember that effective interventions will address the systemic issues identified through your root cause analysis, not just the symptoms. This ensures long-term positive impact rather than merely short-term gains.

Regular monitoring and evaluation are paramount. Continuously assess the effectiveness of your interventions. Track key metrics to gauge the impact of your changes. Regular reviews allow for timely adjustments and course corrections, ensuring progress is maintained. Don't assume your initial interventions will work flawlessly; be prepared to adapt your strategies based on your ongoing assessment of their effectiveness. Consistent monitoring prevents regression and ensures continual improvement.

Finally, foster a culture of safety and continuous improvement. A supportive work environment where staff feel empowered to report errors and near misses is crucial. Open communication and collaborative problem-solving create a proactive culture where safety is valued and continuous improvement is seen as a collaborative effort. Remember to celebrate successes; recognizing achievements fosters positive reinforcement and sustains commitment to ongoing performance enhancement. Positive feedback and recognition build trust and bolster morale. A strong safety culture is not just a policy; it is a mindset that permeates all aspects of the organization. The collaborative culture should facilitate the proactive identification and resolution of safety concerns, ensuring lasting improvements in performance. The collective effort ensures a stronger safety net for all staff and patients. The focus should remain on promoting a culture of mutual respect, where diverse perspectives are valued.

Remember, performance improvement isn't a one-time event; it's an ongoing process. It requires consistent commitment to data-driven decision-making, robust investigation, and adaptive strategies. By embracing these principles, healthcare facilities can achieve significant improvements in safety and quality of care, leading to better outcomes for patients and a more satisfying work environment for staff. Continuous improvement is a marathon, not a sprint, requiring dedication and perseverance, but its rewards are invaluable. This iterative, data-driven approach enhances not only performance, but also trust, engagement, and a shared sense of purpose among the entire healthcare team. Ultimately, it's about a holistic strategy that cultivates a culture focused on providing the best possible patient care, while simultaneously upholding the well-being and development of healthcare professionals.

6.3 Root Cause Analysis

Understanding the root cause of an adverse event, not just its symptoms, is critical for effective prevention. We don't just want to treat the wound; we must identify what caused the patient to fall in the first place. This requires a systematic approach, a methodical journey beyond the immediate observation to the underlying issue. A superficial understanding might lead to temporary fixes, masking the persistent danger. True improvement necessitates deep understanding, a commitment to uncovering the 'why' behind the 'what'. Focusing solely on immediate fixes, without addressing the underlying issues, is like patching a leaking roof with band-aids. Sure, it might temporarily stop the water, but the next rain will bring more problems. You'll be constantly chasing symptoms rather than fixing the core problem. This reactive approach is inefficient and ultimately unsustainable, exhausting resources and frustrating staff. A proactive approach demands a more thorough investigation.

The "five whys" technique, a simple yet powerful tool, guides us through this investigation. By repeatedly asking "why" after each answer, we peel back layers of explanation, progressively revealing deeper causes. For instance, if a patient experienced a medication error, the first "why" might be, "because the wrong dose was administered." The second "why" might then be, "because the label was unclear." Continue asking "why" until you reach the root cause - perhaps an outdated labelling system.

However, the "five whys" is just a starting point. More complex situations require more sophisticated tools. Techniques like the fishbone diagram (Ishikawa diagram) offer a visual framework for brainstorming contributing factors. This method encourages collaborative brainstorming, bringing together diverse perspectives and expertise to identify potential causes, ranging from equipment malfunctions to human error. The collaborative aspect enhances the process, ensuring a more complete picture.

Consider the case of a hospital-acquired infection. A simplistic view might attribute it solely to inadequate hand hygiene. Yet a deeper dive, using a fishbone diagram, might reveal a multitude of contributing factors: insufficient supplies of hand sanitizer, a lack of staff training, poor infection control protocols, inadequately cleaned equipment, or even underlying systemic issues within the hospital's infection control program. Addressing one factor without the others would yield limited success.

Root cause analysis isn't just about identifying problems; it's about building solutions. Once you understand the underlying causes, you can develop targeted interventions to prevent recurrence. It's a crucial step in continuous quality improvement, moving from reactive problem-solving to proactive risk management. The insights gained from this thorough process inform changes in policies, procedures, and training programs.

Remember, the goal isn't to assign blame but to understand the system's vulnerabilities. A culture of blame hinders improvement, while a culture of learning encourages open discussion and constructive solutions. The focus should be on systemic improvements rather than individual failures. This shift in mindset is paramount for sustained progress in patient safety. Effective implementation is key.

Finally, effective implementation of root cause analysis requires clear communication and collaboration. Involving staff at all levels ensures buy-in and fosters a shared commitment to improving safety. Regular review of findings reinforces learning and adaptation, making the entire process dynamic rather than static. This iterative approach to continuous improvement is essential. Implementing the changes is only the beginning of the process. The cycle needs to continue. We must constantly refine our approach and reassess our strategies.

6.4 Continuous Quality Improvement

Continuous quality improvement isn't a single event; it's a journey. Think of it as a continuous cycle of refinement, always striving for better patient outcomes and a safer work environment. It demands a commitment to ongoing monitoring, analysis, and adaptation, not a one-time fix. The ultimate goal is to embed safety into the very fabric of your healthcare system, making it not just a priority, but an inherent part of daily practice. This requires a cultural shift, a collective commitment from every member of the team.

Effective continuous quality improvement hinges on robust data collection. You need reliable, relevant information to pinpoint areas needing attention. This isn't about collecting data for data's sake; it's about gathering specific, measurable information that will inform targeted interventions. Consider using standardized tools to ensure consistency and avoid bias in your data collection methods. Think about patient falls - are they clustered in certain areas? Are certain shifts experiencing more incidents? Analyzing data such as medication errors or hospital-acquired infections in a similar way will reveal patterns and pinpoint potential root causes. Identifying these trends allows you to target your efforts effectively and achieve measurable improvements.

Once you've identified problematic areas, the next step is to understand why these issues are occurring. Root cause analysis, a technique already explored in this book, is critical here. Don't just treat the symptoms; dig deeper to uncover the underlying causes. For instance, if you're seeing a high rate of medication errors, don't simply reprimand the staff involved; investigate the systems and processes that contributed to the errors. Was there inadequate training? Were workflows confusing or overly complex? Were there communication breakdowns? Thoroughly investigating these root causes using tools like the "five whys" or fishbone diagrams will lead to more effective and lasting solutions.

Implementing solutions requires careful planning and execution. It's not enough to simply identify a problem and propose a solution; you need a well-defined plan for implementing that solution. This plan should include clear objectives, timelines, responsibilities, and metrics for evaluating success. Remember, the best solutions are often the simplest and most practical; overly complex interventions can be difficult to implement and sustain. Consider implementing changes gradually, testing them in a small pilot program before rolling them out organization-wide. This approach helps to minimize disruption and allows for adjustments based on feedback from staff and patients.

Once your changes are implemented, the process doesn't end. Continuous monitoring is crucial to assess the effectiveness of your interventions. Are the changes having the desired impact? Are there unintended consequences? Are you seeing improvements in your key metrics? Regular review of your data is essential for identifying any issues or areas that need further refinement. If your interventions are not producing the expected results, don't be afraid to re-evaluate your approach. Flexibility and a willingness to adjust your strategies as needed are key elements of a successful continuous quality improvement process. Remember, it's an iterative process—a continuous cycle of improvement.

Finally, remember that continuous quality improvement is not just about processes and procedures; it's also about people. Engaging your staff in the process is vital for success. When people feel valued and empowered to contribute to safety improvements, they are more likely to be invested in the outcome. Creating a culture of safety, where reporting errors is seen as a learning opportunity rather than a blame-worthy event, is paramount. Encourage open communication, provide adequate training, and celebrate successes to foster a positive and collaborative environment. Ultimately, creating a culture of safety is the foundation for achieving sustainable continuous quality improvement. A culture that values continuous learning, open communication, and the continuous pursuit of better patient outcomes. The journey towards continuous improvement is ongoing. It necessitates sustained efforts, adaptable strategies, and a unified commitment towards a safer healthcare environment. Regularly revisit your processes, and remember that your goal is not merely to meet standards but to consistently exceed them, safeguarding patient well-being and setting the benchmark for excellence within the healthcare landscape.

6.5 Safety Culture Development

A strong safety culture isn't just about policies; it's about a shared belief that safety is paramount. It's a collective commitment woven into the fabric of the healthcare organization, influencing every decision, from the smallest task to the most complex procedure. Building this culture requires a multifaceted approach, demanding consistent effort and dedication from leadership and staff alike.

Open communication is fundamental. This doesn't mean just formal meetings; it requires fostering an environment where individuals feel comfortable voicing concerns, reporting near misses, or identifying potential hazards without fear of retribution. Creating anonymous reporting systems and conducting regular safety huddles can significantly encourage this open dialogue. We need active participation; everyone should feel empowered to contribute to a safer working environment.

Leadership plays a pivotal role in shaping this culture. Leaders must visibly champion safety, not just through words but through actions. Their commitment must be unwavering, demonstrated by actively participating in safety initiatives, allocating sufficient resources, and consistently reinforcing safety expectations. They need to show, not just tell, how safety is a top priority. This includes investing in training, providing necessary equipment, and supporting staff development in safety-related areas.

Effective training is crucial. It's not enough to simply provide mandatory safety training. Instead, healthcare organizations should invest in engaging and interactive training programs that reinforce safe practices and equip staff with the knowledge and skills to manage safety risks effectively. Regular refreshers and scenario-based training—incorporating simulation exercises and real-life case studies—will greatly improve retention and application of the training. The training should go beyond compliance; it should promote a mindset of proactive safety.

Regular audits and feedback mechanisms are essential for continuous improvement. Regular safety audits provide valuable data that helps pinpoint areas needing improvement and assesses the effectiveness of existing safety measures. Feedback from staff, patients, and families should be actively sought and integrated into the improvement process. It allows for a continuous cycle of evaluation and enhancement, preventing complacency and fostering a culture of constant learning.

Incident reporting and investigation should never be viewed as blame-placing exercises. Instead, they represent valuable opportunities to learn from mistakes and improve safety procedures. A thorough investigation that focuses on identifying system failures rather than individual shortcomings will foster a more receptive environment for reporting. We need to make sure the reporting process is straightforward, confidential, and non-punitive, which will encourage prompt reporting. The data collected through this process will shape the organization's safety practices and ultimately improve outcomes.

Beyond formal processes, cultivating a positive and supportive work environment is crucial. A culture where teamwork and mutual respect are valued will naturally lead to improved safety. When staff members feel valued, respected, and heard, they are more likely to contribute actively to safety initiatives. A psychologically safe working environment is, thus, paramount for nurturing a strong safety culture. Empowering staff to take ownership of safety, allowing them to participate in decision-making processes related to safety improvements, greatly enhances engagement.

Finally, celebrating successes and recognizing contributions is key to sustaining the momentum. Highlighting achievements in safety, recognizing individuals or teams who have gone above and beyond, and celebrating milestones will strengthen the collective sense of accomplishment and further reinforce the importance of safety. This positive reinforcement is crucial for motivating staff to continue their commitment to safety. Regular recognition should not be overlooked as it fosters a sense of ownership and pride among the team. Creating a culture of safety isn't merely a checklist; it's a continuous journey. It takes consistent effort, commitment, and collaboration. Yet, the rewards—a safer workplace and improved patient outcomes—are well worth the investment.

7 Future Trends in Healthcare Safety

The integration of artificial intelligence (AI) and machine learning (ML) into healthcare is rapidly transforming safety protocols. AI-powered diagnostic tools can detect subtle abnormalities in medical images far exceeding human capabilities, leading to earlier and more accurate diagnoses. This translates to improved patient outcomes and reduced medical errors. Moreover, AI algorithms can analyze massive datasets of patient information to identify high-risk individuals, allowing for proactive interventions and preventative care. Predictive modeling can forecast potential complications, enabling healthcare professionals to take preemptive measures and ultimately minimize adverse events. This proactive approach, coupled with real-time monitoring capabilities, represents a significant leap forward in patient safety.

Beyond diagnostic applications, AI is revolutionizing medication management. Smart drug delivery systems, guided by AI algorithms, can ensure precise and timely medication administration, minimizing errors and improving adherence. AI-powered systems can also monitor patients remotely, detecting early signs of deterioration and alerting healthcare providers promptly, facilitating timely interventions. These advancements are not only improving the quality of care but also reducing the burden on healthcare professionals, allowing them to focus on more complex tasks.

The rise of telehealth and remote patient monitoring further amplifies the role of technology in ensuring safety. Wearable sensors and connected devices collect vital signs and other physiological data, transmitting information directly to healthcare professionals. This real-time monitoring allows for quick identification of critical events, enabling prompt responses and potentially life-saving interventions. Telehealth platforms facilitate virtual consultations and remote diagnostics, especially beneficial for patients in remote areas or with mobility limitations, improving access to care and ensuring timely interventions. However, cybersecurity measures must be robust to protect sensitive patient data from unauthorized access.

Emerging infectious diseases pose a persistent threat to global health security. Antimicrobial resistance is a growing concern, requiring innovative strategies to combat the spread of resistant pathogens. Advanced diagnostics and rapid pathogen identification tools are crucial for effective infection control. Data analytics and epidemiological modeling play a vital role in predicting outbreaks and guiding public health interventions. Investing in robust surveillance systems and strengthening global collaboration are paramount in mitigating the impact of future pandemics and emerging infections.

The development of novel vaccines and therapeutics is crucial in safeguarding against emerging infectious diseases. Research into innovative vaccine platforms and advanced drug delivery systems is underway, promising faster response times and more effective interventions. Biosecurity measures and enhanced laboratory safety protocols are also essential in preventing accidental release of dangerous pathogens and minimizing the risk of outbreaks. Investing in research and development, coupled with robust public health infrastructure, is vital in combating the challenges posed by emerging infectious diseases.

Furthermore, addressing healthcare disparities and improving access to quality care remains a critical priority. Technology plays a crucial role in overcoming geographical barriers and reducing inequities in healthcare access. Telehealth platforms and mobile health applications can extend healthcare services to underserved communities, ensuring timely and appropriate care for everyone. Equitable access to preventive care and health education programs is essential in reducing health disparities and improving population health outcomes. Initiatives focusing on improving health literacy and promoting preventative measures are crucial in fostering a healthier and safer population.

It is crucial to address ethical implications arising from technological advancements in healthcare. Data privacy and security are paramount, requiring robust regulations and security measures to protect sensitive patient information. Algorithmic bias and fairness in AI-powered systems must be addressed to prevent discriminatory outcomes. Transparency and accountability are essential in ensuring ethical and responsible use of technology in healthcare settings. Open communication and public engagement are crucial in building trust and ensuring that technological advancements benefit all members of society. A collaborative approach among stakeholders, including healthcare providers, policymakers, researchers, and the public, is essential to navigate the complex ethical landscape of future healthcare safety.

The human element remains crucial in maintaining a culture of safety. Investing in training and education for healthcare professionals is vital in fostering a safety-conscious workforce. Promoting open communication and encouraging reporting of near misses and errors are essential in creating a learning environment. A strong safety culture, where reporting errors is encouraged without fear of retribution, is fundamental in preventing future incidents. Continuous improvement initiatives, fueled by data analysis and feedback, are key to refining safety protocols and promoting a just culture within healthcare organizations. Building a culture of safety is a continuous process, requiring active participation and commitment from all stakeholders.

7.1 Technology & Safety

Technology offers incredible opportunities to enhance patient safety and streamline healthcare processes. Consider, for instance, the implementation of electronic health records (EHRs). These systems, when properly utilized, can significantly reduce medication errors through built-in alerts and reminders. They also facilitate better communication between healthcare providers, leading to improved coordination of care and reduced risks of adverse events. However, EHRs also present challenges; the sheer volume of data and the potential for system failures necessitate robust training and ongoing maintenance to maximize their benefits and minimize their drawbacks. Properly implemented, electronic medication administration records (eMARs) can prevent medication errors by providing real-time tracking and verification, a feature especially important for high-alert medications. This technology, coupled with barcode scanning, creates a layered system of checks and balances significantly reducing the potential for human error. Integration of clinical decision support systems (CDSS) into EHRs can further enhance safety by providing alerts and recommendations based on patient-specific data and best practices.

Telemedicine presents another avenue for improved safety, particularly in remote or underserved areas. Patients can receive timely consultations and monitoring, reducing the need for potentially risky travel. Real-time remote patient monitoring (RPM) devices can track vital signs, medication adherence, and other relevant data, enabling early detection of potential problems. This proactive approach allows for timely intervention and prevents the escalation of minor issues into major complications. However, the successful implementation of RPM relies heavily on patient engagement and reliable technology infrastructure. Data security and patient privacy must also be paramount considerations, requiring stringent protocols and adherence to regulations. Furthermore, the integration of RPM data into EHRs is crucial to maintain a comprehensive patient record, providing a holistic view of the patient's health status for seamless care coordination.

Beyond direct patient care, technology plays a crucial role in enhancing hospital infrastructure safety. Smart building technologies can monitor environmental conditions, such as temperature and humidity, optimizing conditions for patient comfort and preventing potential risks related to equipment malfunction or environmental hazards. Real-time location systems (RTLS) can track the location of medical equipment and personnel, improving efficiency and reducing the risk of misplaced items or delayed responses in emergencies. These systems can also assist in fall prevention by tracking patient movement and triggering alerts if a patient leaves their bed or attempts to ambulate without assistance. In addition, automated systems for disinfection and sterilization can significantly reduce the risk of hospital-acquired infections, playing a vital role in infection control measures. It's crucial, however, to acknowledge the need for ongoing investment in system maintenance, robust training programs for staff to ensure their adept utilization, and consideration of potential security vulnerabilities.

Artificial intelligence (AI) holds immense promise for enhancing healthcare safety. AI-powered diagnostic tools can assist clinicians in making more accurate and timely diagnoses, potentially preventing adverse events by identifying problems earlier. AI algorithms can analyze large datasets to identify patterns and predict risks, enabling proactive interventions and resource allocation. However, the responsible development and deployment of AI in healthcare require careful consideration of ethical implications, bias in algorithms, and data privacy concerns. Validation and rigorous testing are essential before widespread adoption to ensure accuracy and reliability. Transparency in the algorithms used, allowing for examination of their methodology and biases, is also critical for building trust and accountability. The ongoing evaluation of AI's performance and continuous improvement through feedback mechanisms will be crucial for long-term success.

The effective integration of technology into healthcare safety requires a multifaceted approach. It necessitates a robust infrastructure, comprehensive training programs for staff, clear protocols, and ongoing system maintenance. Addressing potential security vulnerabilities and data privacy concerns is paramount, ensuring that patient information is protected. Collaboration between healthcare providers, technology developers, and regulatory bodies is crucial to foster innovation and ensure that technological advancements are implemented safely and responsibly. By embracing technology judiciously and thoughtfully, healthcare can significantly improve safety, enhance the quality of care, and ultimately improve patient outcomes. The future of healthcare safety hinges on our ability to leverage technology's potential responsibly and strategically.

7.2 Emerging Infections

The rise of antimicrobial resistance presents a significant challenge. Years of overreliance on antibiotics have fueled the evolution of "superbugs"—bacteria, viruses, fungi, and parasites that defy conventional treatments. These resistant pathogens cause infections that are harder to treat, leading to longer illnesses, higher medical costs, and increased mortality rates. Understanding this evolving landscape is crucial for effective prevention and control. We must focus on responsible antibiotic stewardship, minimizing unnecessary prescriptions, and promoting alternative therapies whenever possible. This requires collaborative efforts between healthcare professionals, researchers, and policymakers. Effective strategies necessitate comprehensive public health initiatives focusing on infection prevention and control. This includes robust surveillance systems to monitor the spread of resistant organisms and the development of novel diagnostic tools for rapid and accurate identification.

Developing new antibiotics and antimicrobial therapies is an urgent priority. However, the pharmaceutical industry faces considerable challenges in this area, including the high cost and long timeframes involved in drug development. Innovative approaches are needed, such as exploring alternative therapeutic strategies, including phage therapy (using viruses to target bacteria) and enhancing the body's natural immune responses. Investing in research and development is vital. Moreover, global collaboration is essential to accelerate the discovery and development of new antimicrobial agents. This collaborative effort will need to involve international organizations, research institutions, and pharmaceutical companies. We need to ensure equitable access to these new therapies when they become available. Equitable distribution is crucial because without it the success of these new treatments will be limited and the problem will worsen. Beyond the development of new treatments, preventing the spread of infections is paramount. Implementing rigorous infection control practices in healthcare settings remains critical. This involves strict adherence to hand hygiene protocols, the appropriate use of personal protective equipment (PPE), and meticulous environmental cleaning. Furthermore, educating healthcare professionals and the public about infection prevention and control is crucial to empower them to take an active role in mitigating the risk of transmission. This education must emphasize the proper use of antibiotics, the importance of vaccination, and the practice of good hygiene. Effective communication strategies are key to effectively convey these messages to diverse populations. These messages must be clear, concise, and culturally appropriate to ensure their effective uptake. Climate change also significantly impacts the emergence of infectious diseases. Changes in temperature and rainfall patterns can alter the distribution and prevalence of disease vectors, such as mosquitoes and ticks. This expansion of vector habitats could lead to the spread of diseases into new geographic areas and increase the incidence of vector-borne illnesses. This shift will require surveillance systems that adapt to account for these changes and adjust strategies to match. Investing in climate-resilient healthcare systems and infrastructure will be crucial to handle potential increases in disease burden in areas facing these changes. We must consider the impact of environmental factors on emerging infections and integrate this understanding into our prevention and control strategies. The relationship between environmental changes and disease will require a comprehensive approach and an interdisciplinary effort.

Finally, strengthening global health security is paramount. This involves enhancing international collaborations to detect and respond to outbreaks rapidly and effectively. The early detection and response to outbreaks is paramount in limiting their spread and minimizing their impact. Establishing effective surveillance systems, developing rapid diagnostic tools, and coordinating international responses are essential components of global health security. Early warning systems and rapid response mechanisms will be crucial to minimizing the impact of future outbreaks. This also requires investing in robust public health infrastructure in countries that may lack sufficient resources to respond effectively to emerging outbreaks. This framework will be crucial in establishing a strong global health security system capable of handling new emerging infections.

www.ingramcontent.com/pod-product-compliance
Lightning Source LLC
LaVergne TN
LVHW022014200926
848481LV00007B/2380
* 9 7 9 8 3 4 9 2 4 6 0 0 5 *